2.024 EDITION

Somatic Therapy for Beginners

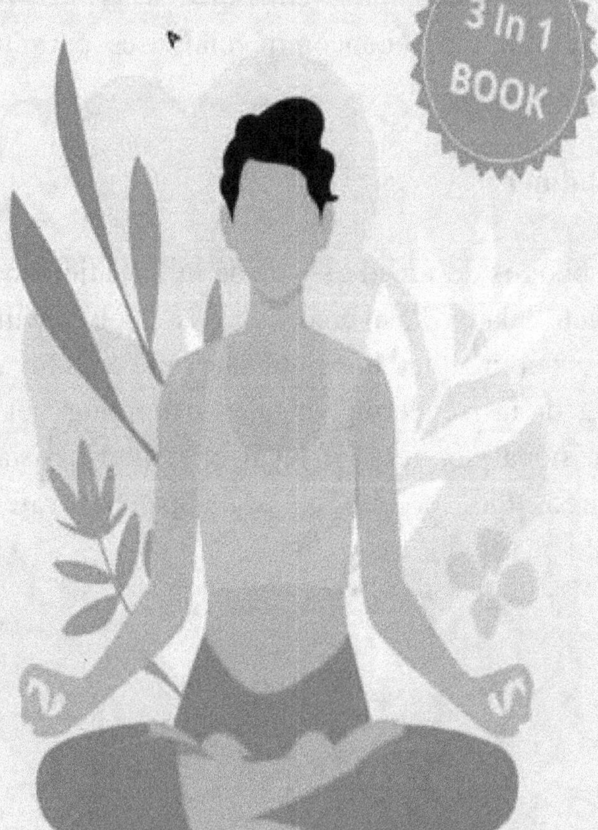

A Practical Guide to Mind-Body Healing for Stress Relief, Trauma Recovery, and Emotional Wellness

RICK TRAVERSE

Disclaimer:

This book is designed to provide information about the subject matter covered. It is sold with the understanding that the publisher and author are not engaged in rendering legal, accounting, or other professional services. If legal or expert assistance is required, the services of a competent professional should be sought.

Table of Contents

Introduction

Somatic therapy is a holistic approach to healing that recognizes the intrinsic connection between the mind and body. This therapeutic modality emphasizes the importance of physical experiences and sensations in our overall well-being. Unlike traditional talk therapies that focus primarily on cognitive processes, somatic therapy incorporates bodily awareness and physical interventions to address psychological issues.

The term "somatic" comes from the Greek word "soma," meaning body. Somatic therapy posits that our bodies hold the imprints of our life experiences, including trauma, stress, and emotions. By tuning into these bodily sensations and experiences, we can access deeper levels of healing and transformation.

Developed in the 1970s by pioneers like Peter Levine and Pat Ogden, somatic therapy has evolved to include various approaches such as Somatic Experiencing, Sensorimotor Psychotherapy, and Hakomi. These methods share a common goal: to help individuals reconnect with their bodies, release stored tension and trauma, and develop greater self-regulation skills.

Somatic therapy is particularly effective in treating issues such as trauma, anxiety, depression, and chronic pain. It provides tools for individuals to become more attuned to their physical sensations, recognize patterns of tension or activation in their bodies, and learn techniques to release and regulate these states.

The Mind-Body Connection

Central to somatic therapy is the understanding that the mind and body are inextricably linked. This connection goes beyond the simple notion that mental stress can cause physical symptoms. Instead, it recognizes that our thoughts, emotions, and physical sensations form a complex, interconnected system.

Neuroscience research supports this view, demonstrating how emotions and thoughts can alter our physiology, and conversely, how physical states can influence our mental and emotional well-being. For example, chronic stress can lead to physical health problems, while adopting certain postures can affect our mood and confidence.

The autonomic nervous system plays a crucial role in this mind-body connection. This system, which regulates many of our involuntary functions, has two main branches: the sympathetic (associated with "fight or flight" responses) and the parasympathetic (associated with "rest and digest" functions). Somatic therapy often focuses on helping individuals balance these systems, promoting a state of relaxed alertness and resilience.

By working with the body, somatic therapy aims to address issues at their root, recognizing that many psychological problems have physical components. This approach can lead to more comprehensive and lasting change, as it addresses not just the cognitive aspects of an issue, but also its physical manifestations and origins.

How to Use This Book

This book is designed to be both a comprehensive guide to somatic therapy and a practical manual for implementing somatic techniques in your daily life. Whether you're a complete beginner or have some experience with body-based practices, you'll find valuable information and exercises to support your healing journey.

The book is divided into three main parts, each focusing on a specific area where somatic therapy can be particularly beneficial: trauma and abuse, anxiety and depression, and stress and burnout. While you may be drawn to one section based on your current needs, we recommend reading the book in its entirety to gain a full understanding of somatic principles and practices.

As you read, we encourage you to approach the material with curiosity and self-compassion. Somatic work can sometimes bring up intense emotions or sensations. It's important to go at your own pace and respect your body's limits. If at any point you feel overwhelmed, take a break or seek support from a qualified professional.

Remember, this book is a tool for self-discovery and healing, but it's not a substitute for professional therapy. If you're dealing with severe trauma, mental health issues, or any medical conditions, consult with a healthcare provider before starting any new therapeutic practices.

By engaging with the concepts and exercises in this book, you're taking an important step towards greater body awareness, emotional regulation, and overall well-being. Welcome to the transformative world of somatic therapy.

PART I

SOMATIC THERAPY FOR TRAUMA AND ABUSE

This section delves into the application of somatic therapy for healing trauma and abuse. Trauma, whether acute or chronic, leaves lasting imprints on the body and nervous system. Somatic approaches offer unique and effective ways to address these deep-seated issues by working directly with the body's stored experiences.

We'll explore how trauma manifests physically, the neurobiology of trauma responses, and specific somatic techniques for trauma resolution. This part also covers the importance of safety, pacing, and self-regulation in trauma work. Through case studies and practical exercises, you'll gain insights into how somatic therapy can facilitate healing, restore a sense of safety in the body, and promote resilience in trauma survivors.

Chapter 1:

Understanding Trauma and Abuse

Trauma and abuse are complex experiences that can profoundly affect an individual's well-being. Trauma refers to deeply distressing or disturbing events that overwhelm one's ability to cope. It can result from a single incident, such as a car accident or natural disaster, or from prolonged exposure to stressful situations, like warfare or chronic neglect. Abuse, on the other hand, involves deliberate acts of harm or mistreatment by one person towards another.

It can take various forms:

1. Physical abuse: Inflicting bodily harm or injury
2. Emotional abuse: Persistent criticism, humiliation, or manipulation
3. Sexual abuse: Non-consensual sexual acts or exploitation
4. Verbal abuse: Using words to control, belittle, or intimidate
5. Financial abuse: Controlling or exploiting someone's financial resources

Both trauma and abuse can occur at any age and have lasting impacts on an individual's mental and physical health.

The Impact on Mind and Body

Trauma and abuse affect not only the mind but also leave lasting imprints on the body. Understanding this dual impact is crucial for effective healing.

Mental Impact:
- Post-Traumatic Stress Disorder (PTSD): Characterized by intrusive memories, hypervigilance, and avoidance behaviors
- Depression: Persistent feelings of sadness, hopelessness, and loss of interest in activities
- Anxiety: Excessive worry, fear, and difficulty relaxing
- Dissociation: Feeling detached from oneself or one's surroundings
- Low self-esteem: Negative self-perception and lack of confidence
- Trust issues: Difficulty forming or maintaining relationships

Physical Impact:
- Chronic pain: Persistent discomfort in various parts of the body
- Sleep disturbances: Insomnia or nightmares

- Digestive issues: Irritable bowel syndrome or other gastrointestinal problems
- Cardiovascular problems: High blood pressure or heart disease
- Weakened immune system: Increased susceptibility to illness
- Altered stress response: Hyperactive or underactive stress hormones

The body often holds the memory of trauma even when the conscious mind has suppressed it. This physical retention can manifest as tension, pain, or unexplained physical symptoms.

How Somatic Therapy Can Help

Somatic therapy offers a unique approach to healing trauma and abuse by addressing both the mental and physical aspects of these experiences. Here's how it can be beneficial:

1. Body awareness: Somatic therapy helps individuals reconnect with their bodies, often after years of dissociation or numbness. This increased awareness allows for the identification and release of stored trauma.
2. Nervous system regulation: Through various techniques, somatic therapy aids in balancing the autonomic nervous system, helping individuals move out of the "fight, flight, or freeze" response that often persists after trauma.

3. Release of stored tension: Physical exercises and touch-based techniques can help release muscle tension and physical patterns related to trauma.
4. Emotional processing: By focusing on bodily sensations, somatic therapy provides a safe way to process emotions that may be too overwhelming to approach cognitively.
5. Empowerment: Somatic practices help individuals regain a sense of control over their bodies and responses, which is often compromised in trauma and abuse.
6. Mindfulness: Somatic therapy incorporates mindfulness techniques, helping individuals stay present and grounded, rather than being caught in past traumatic memories.
7. Integration of experiences: By working with both body and mind, somatic therapy facilitates the integration of traumatic experiences into one's life narrative in a healthier way.
8. Improved relationships: As individuals become more attuned to their own bodies and emotions, they often experience improved relationships and social connections.

Somatic therapy doesn't require individuals to relive or extensively recount their traumatic experiences. Instead, it focuses on present-moment bodily sensations and experiences, making it a gentler approach for many trauma survivors.
In the following chapters, we'll explore specific somatic techniques that can be used to address trauma

and abuse, helping you on your journey towards healing and resilience. Remember, while these techniques can be powerful tools for self-help, it's important to work with a qualified professional when dealing with severe trauma or abuse.

Chapter 2:

Somatic Techniques for Trauma Healing

This chapter introduces practical somatic techniques that can aid in healing from trauma. These methods focus on reconnecting with your body, increasing awareness, and releasing stored tension. While these exercises can be powerful tools for self-help, individuals with severe trauma should practice them under the guidance of a trained professional.

A. Grounding Exercises

Grounding techniques help anchor you in the present moment, counteracting the dissociation often experienced in trauma. These exercises engage your senses and physical awareness to create a sense of safety and stability.

1. The 5-4-3-2-1 Technique:
   - Identify 5 things you can see
   - Notice 4 things you can touch
   - Recognize 3 things you can hear
   - Acknowledge 2 things you can smell

o   Name 1 thing you can taste

This exercise redirects attention to your immediate environment, engaging multiple senses.

2. Feet-to-Ground:
    o   Stand or sit with your feet flat on the floor
    o   Focus on the sensation of your feet touching the ground
    o   Imagine roots growing from your feet into the earth
    o   Breathe deeply, visualizing stability flowing up through these roots

3. Object Focus:
    o   Choose a small object you can hold
    o   Examine its texture, weight, temperature, and any other physical properties
    o   Describe these qualities to yourself, focusing solely on the object

Practice these exercises regularly, especially when feeling overwhelmed or disconnected.

B. Body Scanning and Awareness

Body scanning cultivates a deeper awareness of physical sensations, helping you recognize and address areas of tension or discomfort.

Basic Body Scan:
1. Lie down in a comfortable position
2. Close your eyes and take several deep breaths

3. Begin at your toes, focusing your attention on any sensations present
4. Slowly move your focus upward through your body, part by part
5. Notice areas of tension, temperature, or other sensations without judgment
6. If you encounter areas of discomfort, breathe into them, imagining tension releasing

Practice this scan daily, ideally for 10-15 minutes. Over time, you'll develop greater bodily awareness and the ability to release tension consciously.

Enhanced Body Awareness Exercise:
1. Stand with your eyes closed
2. Shift your weight slightly from side to side, then front to back
3. Notice how these small movements affect different parts of your body
4. Pay attention to which muscles engage and how your balance adjusts
5. Gradually increase the range of motion, maintaining awareness of bodily sensations

This exercise enhances proprioception (awareness of body position) and can help reestablish a sense of control over your physical self.

Trauma Release Exercises (TRE)

Trauma Release Exercises, developed by Dr. David Berceli, involve inducing mild tremors in the body to release deep muscular tension associated with trauma.

Basic TRE Sequence:

1. Lie on your back with knees bent, feet flat on the floor
2. Slowly bring your feet together, allowing knees to fall outward
3. Lift your hips slightly, creating an arch in your lower back
4. Hold this position for 1-2 minutes, or until you feel mild muscle fatigue
5. Slowly lower your hips and allow your legs to straighten
6. Notice any trembling or shaking that occurs in your legs or pelvis
7. Allow this trembling to continue for 5-15 minutes, or until it naturally subsides
8. Rest for a few minutes afterward, noticing any changes in your body

Important notes:

- Start with short sessions (5-10 minutes) and gradually increase duration
- If tremors feel too intense, return your feet to the floor to stop them
- Avoid TRE if you have recent injuries, are pregnant, or have certain medical conditions

These exercises can release deep-seated tension and trauma stored in the body. However, they may also bring up intense emotions. Always prioritize your comfort and safety, and don't hesitate to seek professional guidance.

Regular practice of these somatic techniques can significantly aid your trauma healing journey. They offer practical tools for managing symptoms, increasing body awareness, and releasing stored tension. Remember to approach these exercises with patience and self-compassion, allowing your body the time it needs to heal.

Chapter 3:

Addressing Dissociation and Flashbacks

Dissociation and flashbacks are common experiences for individuals who have endured trauma. Dissociation is a disconnection from one's thoughts, feelings, memories, or sense of identity. It's a protective mechanism that can become problematic when it persists beyond the traumatic event. Signs of dissociation include:

1. Feeling detached from your body or surroundings
2. Experiencing the world as unreal or dreamlike
3. Losing track of time or experiencing time distortions
4. Feeling emotionally numb or disconnected
5. Having difficulty remembering specific events or periods

To recognize dissociation, practice regular check-ins with your body and environment. Ask yourself:
- Can I feel my feet on the ground?
- Am I aware of my surroundings?
- Can I identify and name my current emotions?
- Do I feel present in my body?

Techniques to Stay Present

These somatic techniques can help you remain grounded and present:

1. Body Tapping:
   o Use your fingertips to gently tap different parts of your body
   o Start with your arms, then legs, torso, and face
   o Focus on the sensation of touch to reconnect with your physical self
2. Temperature Contrast:
   o Hold an ice cube in one hand and a warm object in the other
   o Alternate your focus between the two sensations
   o This stark contrast helps anchor you in the present moment
3. Sensory Engagement:
   o Carry small objects with distinct textures (e.g., a smooth stone, a rough piece of bark)
   o When feeling disconnected, touch these objects and focus on their unique properties
   o Describe the sensations to yourself in detail
4. Rhythmic Breathing:
   o Inhale for a count of 4, hold for 4, exhale for 4, hold for 4
   o Repeat this pattern, focusing on the physical sensations of breathing
   o This technique regulates the nervous system and promotes presence

5. Progressive Muscle Relaxation:
   - Tense and then relax each muscle group in your body
   - Start from your toes and work up to your face
   - This exercise increases body awareness and releases tension

Managing Flashbacks Somatically

Flashbacks are intense, vivid memories of a traumatic event that feel as if they're happening in the present. Somatic approaches can help manage these distressing experiences:

1. Orienting Technique:
   - Look around the room and name objects you see
   - Touch nearby surfaces and describe their textures
   - This helps your brain recognize that you're in the present, not the past
2. Grounding Pose:
   - Sit in a chair with your feet flat on the floor
   - Press your feet down and feel the solid ground beneath you
   - Place your hands on your thighs and apply gentle pressure
   - Focus on these points of contact to anchor yourself in the present
3. Body Boundaries:
   - Use your hands to firmly trace the outline of your body

- Start at your head and work down to your feet
- This reinforces your physical boundaries and present-moment existence

4. Bilateral Stimulation:
- Alternately tap your right and left knees or shoulders
- This rhythmic, side-to-side stimulation can help integrate traumatic memories

5. Safe Place Visualization with Somatic Focus:
- Imagine a place where you feel completely safe
- Engage all your senses in this visualization
- Pay particular attention to how your body feels in this safe place
- When the flashback subsides, slowly bring your awareness back to the present

6. Temperature Regulation:
- Keep a cold pack and a heating pad accessible
- During a flashback, alternate between these temperature extremes
- Focus on the physical sensations to redirect your attention

Remember, these techniques may take practice to become effective. Be patient with yourself and consistently apply these methods. If flashbacks persist or severely impact your daily life, consult a trauma-informed therapist for additional support.

By incorporating these somatic techniques into your daily routine and using them when dissociation or flashbacks occur, you can gradually increase your ability to stay present and manage trauma-related symptoms. This somatic approach helps rebuild the connection between mind and body, fostering resilience and healing.

Chapter 4:

Rebuilding Safety and Boundaries

Trauma and abuse often compromise one's sense of safety and personal boundaries. This chapter focuses on somatic approaches to rebuild these essential aspects of well-being.

A. Creating a Safe Space

A safe space serves as a foundation for healing and self-exploration. It's both a physical location and an internal state of being.

Physical Safe Space:
1. Choose a quiet, private area in your home
2. Personalize it with comforting items (e.g., soft blankets, calming artwork)
3. Engage multiple senses:
   - Sight: Use soft, warm lighting
   - Sound: Play soothing music or nature sounds
   - Smell: Incorporate calming scents like lavender or vanilla

- Touch: Include textures that feel comforting to you

Internal Safe Space Exercise:
1. Sit or lie comfortably in your physical safe space
2. Close your eyes and take several deep breaths
3. Visualize a place where you feel completely safe and at peace
4. Engage all your senses in this visualization
5. Notice how your body feels in this safe place
6. Create a physical gesture (e.g., placing your hand over your heart) to anchor this feeling
7. Practice accessing this internal safe space daily, using your anchor gesture

B. Boundary-Setting Exercises

Boundaries are crucial for self-protection and healthy relationships. These somatic exercises help reinforce your personal boundaries:
1. Body Bubble Visualization:
   - Stand with your eyes closed
   - Imagine a protective bubble surrounding your body
   - Visualize this bubble expanding and contracting with your breath
   - Practice maintaining this bubble as you move around
2. Physical Boundary Practice:
   - Stand facing a partner (or imagine one)

- Take a step forward until you feel slightly uncomfortable
- Notice the physical sensations in your body
- Step back until you feel at ease again
- Repeat this process, paying attention to your body's signals

3. Embodied "No" Exercise:
   - Stand with feet hip-width apart
   - Extend your arm in front of you, palm facing out
   - Say "No" firmly while pushing your hand forward
   - Notice the sensations in your body as you do this
   - Practice varying the intensity of your "No"

4. Personal Space Mapping:
   - Use chalk or tape to create concentric circles around you
   - Label each circle (e.g., intimate, personal, social, public)
   - Practice allowing different people into different zones
   - Pay attention to your bodily responses as you do this

Self-Defense and Empowerment Practices

These practices aim to increase your sense of personal power and ability to protect yourself:

1. Grounding Stance:
   - Stand with feet shoulder-width apart
   - Bend your knees slightly
   - Engage your core muscles
   - Feel your connection to the ground
   - Practice this stance daily to embody stability and strength
2. Power Posing:
   - Stand tall with your feet apart and hands on your hips
   - Hold this pose for two minutes
   - Notice how it affects your mood and confidence
   - Incorporate this pose into your daily routine
3. Vocal Empowerment:
   - Practice speaking from your diaphragm
   - Start with humming, then progress to vowel sounds
   - Finally, practice saying "No" and "Stop" with a strong, clear voice
   - Notice how using your voice affects your body
4. Basic Self-Defense Moves:
   - Learn and practice simple techniques like:
     - Palm heel strike
     - Knee strike
     - Elbow strike
   - Focus on the body mechanics and how they make you feel

- Remember, the goal is empowerment, not aggression

5. Tension and Release:
   - Tense all the muscles in your body for 5 seconds
   - Release the tension quickly
   - Notice the sensation of relaxation that follows
   - This exercise helps you recognize and release tension in high-stress situations

6. Mindful Movement:
   - Practice slow, deliberate movements (e.g., tai chi or slow martial arts forms)
   - Focus on each movement's power and intention
   - This cultivates body awareness and a sense of control

Implementation Tips:
- Start slowly and be patient with yourself
- Practice these exercises regularly, even when you feel safe
- If any exercise causes distress, stop and return to your safe space
- Consider working with a trauma-informed self-defense instructor for personalized guidance

By consistently practicing these somatic techniques, you can gradually rebuild your sense of safety and strengthen your personal boundaries. Remember, this process takes time and patience. Celebrate small victories and be compassionate with yourself as you progress on this healing journey.

As you become more attuned to your body's signals and more confident in setting and maintaining boundaries, you'll likely find that your overall sense of safety and empowerment increases both in your internal world and in your interactions with others.

Chapter 5:

Healing Touch and Intimacy after Abuse

This chapter addresses the challenges of reestablishing healthy touch and intimacy following experiences of abuse. It's crucial to approach this topic with patience, self-compassion, and respect for individual boundaries.

Consensual Touch Exercises

These exercises aim to reintroduce positive, safe touch experiences. Always prioritize consent and personal comfort.

1. Self-Touch Exploration:
   - Begin with self-touch to reconnect with your body
   - Use different pressures, textures, and temperatures
   - Notice physical sensations without judgment
   - Practice saying "yes" or "no" to different types of touch
2. Boundary Mapping:
   - Use a body outline drawing

- Color areas where touch feels comfortable (green), uncertain (yellow), or uncomfortable (red)
  - Update this map regularly to track progress
3. Hand-on-Hand Exercise (with a trusted partner):
  - Sit facing your partner
  - Place your hand palm-up between you
  - Have your partner slowly move their hand towards yours
  - Say "stop" when you feel any discomfort
  - Practice finding the distance that feels safe
4. Mindful Massage (solo or partnered):
  - Focus on one body part (e.g., hand, foot)
  - Apply lotion or oil slowly and mindfully
  - Pay attention to sensations, temperature, and pressure
  - If partnered, communicate preferences clearly
5. Breath Synchronization:
  - Sit back-to-back with a partner
  - Focus on your own breath, then try to synchronize with your partner
  - This creates intimacy without direct touch

Rebuilding Trust in Relationships

Trust is fundamental for healthy intimacy. These practices help rebuild trust with yourself and others.
1. Trust Barometer:
  - Regularly check in with your body's responses in various situations

o Notice physical signs of trust (relaxation) or distrust (tension)
   o Use this awareness to guide your decisions in relationships
2. Transparent Communication Practice:
   o With a trusted friend or partner, take turns sharing:
       ■ Current feelings
       ■ Physical sensations
       ■ Needs or boundaries
   o Practice active listening without judgment
3. Gradual Exposure:
   o Create a hierarchy of intimate actions (e.g., eye contact, holding hands, hugging)
   o Slowly progress through this list at your own pace
   o Always respect your current boundaries
4. Body Scan for Emotional Awareness:
   o Regularly perform body scans to identify emotions
   o Link physical sensations to specific emotions
   o Share these insights with trusted individuals to deepen connections
5. Collaborative Boundary Setting:
   o With a partner, discuss and agree on physical and emotional boundaries
   o Regularly revisit and adjust these boundaries
   o Practice respectfully asserting and hearing boundaries

Somatic Sexuality Practices

These practices focus on reconnecting with your body's capacity for pleasure and intimate connection. Approach them at your own pace.

1. Sensate Focus:
    - Explore your body with curiosity, not sexual intent
    - Notice various sensations: pressure, temperature, texture
    - Gradually include a partner if comfortable, maintaining communication
2. Mindful Self-Pleasure:
    - Explore self-touch with a focus on pleasure, not performance
    - Pay attention to your body's responses
    - Practice saying "yes" to enjoyable sensations
3. Trauma-Sensitive Yoga:
    - Engage in gentle yoga practices focusing on:
        - Grounding
        - Body awareness
        - Breath work
    - This helps reconnect with your body in a non-sexual context
4. Pelvic Floor Awareness:
    - Learn to identify and relax your pelvic floor muscles
    - Practice tensing and releasing these muscles
    - This increases body awareness and can enhance sexual experiences
5. Embodied Consent Practice:

- With a partner, take turns initiating non-sexual touch
- Practice saying "yes," "no," or "maybe" based on your authentic body response
- Respect each other's responses without question

6. Somatic Resourcing:
- Identify physical sensations that feel safe and pleasurable
- Use these as "resources" during intimate experiences
- If triggered, focus on these pleasant sensations to re-center yourself

Implementation Guidelines:

- Always prioritize your comfort and safety
- Progress at your own pace; there's no timeline for healing
- It's okay and normal to have setbacks; be patient with yourself
- Consider working with a trauma-informed sex therapist for personalized guidance
- Communicate openly with partners about your needs and boundaries
- Remember that healing is possible and you deserve healthy, joyful intimacy

By consistently practicing these somatic approaches, you can gradually reconnect with your body, rebuild trust, and rediscover your capacity for healthy touch and intimacy. This journey requires patience, self-compassion, and often the support of trusted individuals or professionals. Remember that every small step forward is a significant achievement in your healing process.

PART II:

SOMATIC THERAPY FOR ANXIETY AND DEPRESSION

This section explores the application of somatic therapy in addressing anxiety and depression. While these conditions are often treated primarily through cognitive approaches, somatic therapy offers a complementary bodily perspective that can enhance healing and management of symptoms.

We'll examine how anxiety and depression manifest in the body, the role of the nervous system in these conditions, and specific somatic techniques for relief. This part covers grounding practices, embodied emotional regulation, and movement-based interventions. Through practical exercises and case studies, you'll learn how to use somatic awareness to interrupt anxious or depressive patterns, cultivate resilience, and foster a greater sense of ease in both body and mind.

Chapter 6:

The Somatic Experience of Anxiety and Depression

This chapter explores the bodily manifestations of anxiety and depression, emphasizing the intricate connection between mental states and physical experiences. Understanding these somatic aspects is crucial for effective treatment and self-management.

Physical Symptoms of Anxiety and Depression

Anxiety and depression, while often considered mental health conditions, have profound effects on the body. Recognizing these physical symptoms is key to early intervention and holistic treatment.

Anxiety-related physical symptoms:
1. Increased heart rate and palpitations
2. Rapid, shallow breathing
3. Muscle tension, particularly in the neck, shoulders, and jaw
4. Gastrointestinal distress (nausea, stomachaches, diarrhea)
5. Excessive sweating

6. Trembling or shaking
7. Fatigue
8. Sleep disturbances
9. Headaches
10. Dizziness or lightheadedness

Depression-related physical symptoms:
1. Persistent fatigue and low energy
2. Changes in sleep patterns (insomnia or hypersomnia)
3. Appetite changes leading to weight loss or gain
4. Psychomotor retardation (slowed movements and speech)
5. Unexplained aches and pains
6. Digestive problems
7. Decreased libido
8. Weakened immune system
9. Heavy feeling in limbs
10. Changes in posture (e.g., slumped shoulders)

It's important to note that individuals may experience these symptoms differently, and some may have symptoms of both anxiety and depression simultaneously.

The Nervous System's Role

The autonomic nervous system plays a crucial role in the physical manifestations of anxiety and depression. This system has two main branches:
1. Sympathetic Nervous System (SNS):
   - Often called the "fight or flight" system

- o Activated during stress and anxiety
- o Increases heart rate, breathing rate, and muscle tension
- o Releases stress hormones like cortisol and adrenaline

2. Parasympathetic Nervous System (PNS):
   - o Known as the "rest and digest" system
   - o Promotes relaxation and recovery
   - o Slows heart rate, deepens breathing, and promotes digestion

In anxiety, the SNS is often overactive, leading to persistent physical arousal. In depression, there may be an imbalance between the SNS and PNS, contributing to the physical symptoms of lethargy and disrupted bodily functions.

Understanding this nervous system involvement helps explain why somatic approaches, which often focus on nervous system regulation, can be effective in treating anxiety and depression.

Somatic Markers and Emotional Awareness

Somatic markers are bodily sensations associated with emotional states. They serve as internal cues that guide decision-making and emotional processing. Developing awareness of these markers is a key aspect of somatic therapy for anxiety and depression.

Examples of somatic markers:

- A "knot" in the stomach during anxiety
- Heaviness in the chest associated with sadness
- Tension in the jaw linked to anger or frustration

The process of identifying and understanding somatic markers involves:

1. Body Scanning:
   - Regularly check in with your body
   - Notice areas of tension, discomfort, or other sensations
   - Observe without judgment
2. Emotion-Sensation Linking:
   - When you identify an emotion, pay attention to accompanying physical sensations
   - Over time, you may notice patterns (e.g., anxiety always causes shoulder tension)
3. Journaling:
   - Keep a log of emotions and their physical manifestations
   - This can help identify patterns and increase body awareness
4. Mindfulness Practices:
   - Engage in mindfulness meditation to enhance overall body awareness
   - This can improve your ability to detect subtle somatic markers
5. Somatic Tracking:
   - When experiencing an emotion, track how it moves through your body
   - Notice any changes in intensity or location of physical sensations

Developing awareness of somatic markers offers several benefits:

- Early detection of anxiety or depressive episodes
- Improved emotional regulation
- Enhanced self-understanding
- More effective communication about emotional states
- Better-informed decision-making based on bodily wisdom

Practical Exercise: Somatic Marker Mapping

1. Draw an outline of a human body
2. Throughout a week, note where you feel sensations related to different emotions
3. Use colors to represent different emotions (e.g., red for anger, blue for sadness)
4. Review your map regularly to identify patterns in your somatic experiences

By understanding the physical symptoms of anxiety and depression, the role of the nervous system, and the concept of somatic markers, you lay a foundation for more effective management of these conditions. This knowledge empowers you to recognize early warning signs, implement targeted interventions, and develop a more nuanced understanding of your emotional experiences. In the following chapters, we'll explore specific somatic techniques to address these physical manifestations and promote overall well-being.

Chapter 7:

Breath and Movement for Anxiety Relief

This chapter explores powerful somatic techniques that utilize breath and movement to alleviate anxiety. These practices aim to regulate the nervous system, reduce physical tension, and promote a sense of calm and control.

Diaphragmatic Breathing Techniques

Diaphragmatic breathing, also known as belly breathing, is a fundamental skill for managing anxiety. It activates the parasympathetic nervous system, promoting relaxation and reducing stress.

Basic Diaphragmatic Breathing:
1. Sit or lie comfortably, placing one hand on your chest and the other on your belly.
2. Inhale slowly through your nose, allowing your belly to expand while keeping your chest relatively still.
3. Exhale slowly through pursed lips, feeling your belly fall.

4. Repeat for 5-10 minutes, focusing on the movement of your breath.

Advanced Techniques:
1. Box Breathing:
    o Inhale for a count of 4
    o Hold the breath for 4
    o Exhale for 4
    o Hold the empty lungs for 4
    o Repeat this cycle for 5-10 minutes
2. 4-7-8 Breathing:
    o Inhale quietly through the nose for 4 counts
    o Hold the breath for 7 counts
    o Exhale forcefully through the mouth for 8 counts
    o Repeat this cycle 4 times
3. Resonant Breathing:
    o Inhale for 5 seconds
    o Exhale for 5 seconds
    o Maintain this rhythm for 5 minutes
    o This creates a 10-second breathing cycle, which can help synchronize heart rate variability

Implement these techniques daily, especially during moments of heightened anxiety. With practice, they become powerful tools for quick anxiety relief.

Progressive Muscle Relaxation

Progressive Muscle Relaxation (PMR) reduces physical tension associated with anxiety. It involves systematically tensing and relaxing different muscle groups.

Basic PMR Routine:
1. Find a comfortable position, either sitting or lying down.
2. Begin with your toes. Tense the muscles as tightly as possible for 5 seconds.
3. Release the tension suddenly and completely. Notice the feeling of relaxation for 15 seconds.
4. Move to the next muscle group (e.g., calves, thighs, buttocks, abdomen, chest, arms, hands, neck, face).
5. Repeat the process for each muscle group, moving up the body.

Advanced PMR Techniques:
1. Body Scan PMR:
   - Instead of tensing muscles, simply focus your attention on each area.
   - Notice any tension and imagine it melting away as you exhale.
2. Visualization-Enhanced PMR:
   - As you release each muscle group, visualize tension flowing out of your body.
   - Imagine it as a color or substance leaving through your fingertips or toes.
3. Abbreviated PMR:
   - Group larger areas together (e.g., entire leg, entire arm) for a quicker session.
   - Useful for on-the-go relaxation.

Practice PMR daily, preferably at the same time, to build a relaxation habit. Over time, you'll become more aware of muscle tension and more skilled at releasing it.

Yoga and Qi Gong for Anxiety

Both yoga and qi gong combine breath, movement, and mindfulness, making them excellent practices for anxiety management.

Yoga for Anxiety:
1. Child's Pose (Balasana):
   - Kneel on the floor, sit back on your heels, and fold forward.
   - Rest your forehead on the ground and extend arms forward or alongside your body.
   - Hold for 1-5 minutes, focusing on deep, slow breaths.
2. Standing Forward Bend (Uttanasana):
   - Stand with feet hip-width apart, fold forward from the hips.
   - Let head and arms hang heavy. Bend knees if needed.
   - Hold for 30 seconds to 1 minute, feeling tension release from the spine.
3. Legs-Up-the-Wall Pose (Viparita Karani):
   - Lie on your back with legs extended up a wall.

- Stay for 5-15 minutes, focusing on slow, deep breathing.

4. Alternate Nostril Breathing (Nadi Shodhana):
   - Use your right thumb to close your right nostril.
   - Inhale through the left nostril, then close it with your ring finger.
   - Open and exhale through the right nostril.
   - Inhale right, close, exhale left.
   - Continue this pattern for 5-10 cycles.

Qi Gong for Anxiety:

1. Shaking Practice:
   - Stand with feet shoulder-width apart.
   - Gently bounces, allowing the movement to travel up your body.
   - Shake arms, shoulders, and head loosely.
   - Continue for 2-5 minutes, then stand still and notice the sensations in your body.
2. Pushing Mountains:
   - Stand with feet hip-width apart.
   - Inhale, raising arms in front of you to shoulder height.
   - Exhale, pushing palms forward as if gently pushing a mountain.
   - Inhale, drawing hands back to the starting position.
   - Repeat 9 times, coordinating breath with movement.
3. Gathering Earth Energy:
   - Stand with feet wider than hip-width.

- o Bend knees and lower hands toward the ground, palms facing down.
- o Inhale, slowly rising and drawing hands up the centerline of your body.
- o When hands reach chest height, separate them and push up toward the sky.
- o Exhale, lowering hands back down to starting position.
- o Repeat 9 times, focusing on the flow of energy.

Incorporate these yoga and qi gong practices into your daily routine. Even 10-15 minutes can significantly impact anxiety levels. Remember to move mindfully and respect your body's limits.

By consistently practicing these breath and movement techniques, you can develop a powerful toolkit for managing anxiety. These somatic approaches not only provide immediate relief but also foster long-term resilience against stress and anxiety. Experiment with different techniques to find what works best for you, and remember that regular practice is key to experiencing lasting benefits.

Chapter 8:

Embodied Practices for Depression

This chapter explores somatic approaches that engage the body to alleviate symptoms of depression. These practices aim to increase energy, improve mood, and foster a sense of connection and vitality.

Movement Therapy and Dance

Movement therapy and dance can be powerful tools for managing depression, as they combine physical activity, emotional expression, and social connection. Benefits of Movement Therapy:

- Increases endorphin production
- Improves body image and self-esteem
- Provides an outlet for emotional expression
- Enhances mind-body connection

Practical Movement Exercises:
1. Authentic Movement:
   - Find a safe, quiet space

- Close your eyes and listen to your body's impulses
  - Allow yourself to move freely, following these impulses
  - Practice for 5-15 minutes daily
2. Expressive Dance:
  - Choose music that resonates with your current emotional state
  - Move freely to the music, expressing your feelings through movement
  - Experiment with different qualities of movement (e.g., sharp, fluid, heavy, light)
3. Body Part Isolation:
  - Focus on moving one body part at a time (e.g., just your hands, then arms, then shoulders)
  - Notice how each movement affects your mood and energy
4. Mirroring Exercise (with a partner):
  - Stand facing your partner
  - Take turns leading slow, deliberate movements
  - The other person mirrors these movements exactly
  - Switch roles after 2-3 minutes
5. Rhythm and Percussion:
  - Use simple percussion instruments or body percussion (clapping, stomping)
  - Create rhythms that express your emotional state
  - Gradually shift to more uplifting rhythms

Incorporate these practices into your routine, starting with just 5-10 minutes daily. Gradually increase duration as you become more comfortable with the exercises.

Forest Bathing and Nature Connection

Engaging with nature can significantly impact depression symptoms, reducing stress and promoting a sense of calm and connection.

Forest Bathing (Shinrin-yoku) Technique:

1. Find a natural area, ideally a forest or wooded park
2. Leave behind your phone and other distractions
3. Walk slowly, allowing your senses to guide you
4. Pause often to observe your surroundings
5. Engage all your senses:
    - Notice the colors and patterns of leaves and bark
    - Listen to bird songs, rustling leaves, or flowing water
    - Feel the textures of trees, rocks, or plants
    - Smell the earthy scents of soil and vegetation
    - Taste the freshness of the air

Nature Connection Practices:
1. Grounding Exercise:

- o Find a safe outdoor spot and remove your shoes
    - o Stand or walk barefoot on natural surfaces (grass, sand, soil)
    - o Focus on the sensations in your feet, imagining roots growing into the earth
2. Cloud Watching:
    - o Lie on your back and observe the clouds
    - o Notice shapes, movements, and changing patterns
    - o Allow your mind to wander and daydream
3. Nature Art:
    - o Collect natural materials (leaves, pebbles, twigs)
    - o Create a small piece of art, focusing on the process rather than the result
    - o Leave your creation for others to discover
4. Plant Care:
    - o Grow indoor plants or tend to a small garden
    - o Engage mindfully in watering, pruning, and nurturing your plants
    - o Observe their growth and changes over time

Aim to spend at least 20 minutes in nature daily, even if it's just sitting in a local park or tending to houseplants.

Posture and Mood Connection

Our physical posture can significantly influence our emotional state. By consciously adjusting our posture, we can positively impact our mood and energy levels.

Posture Awareness Exercise:

1. Stand in front of a mirror or ask a friend to observe you
2. Notice your habitual posture:
   - Is your head forward or aligned with your spine?
   - Are your shoulders rounded or pulled back?
   - Is your chest open or collapsed?
   - Is your spine straight or curved?
   - Are your knees locked or slightly bent?

Mood-Enhancing Posture Practices:

1. Power Posing:
   - Stand with feet hip-width apart
   - Place hands on hips or raise arms in a V-shape
   - Hold for 2 minutes, breathing deeply
   - Notice any shifts in your mood or energy
2. Heart-Opening Stretch:
   - Interlace fingers behind your back
   - Gently pull your hands down and away from your body
   - Lift your chest and chin slightly
   - Hold for 30 seconds, breathing deeply
3. Smile Muscle Activation:
   - Gently lift the corners of your mouth
   - Hold this subtle smile for 1 minute
   - Notice any changes in your emotional state
4. Tension Release Sequence:

- Exaggerate a "depressed" posture (slumped shoulders, downcast eyes)
  - Hold for 10 seconds, noticing how it feels
  - Slowly shift to an upright, open posture
  - Notice the contrast and the shift in your mood
5. Walking Tall:
  - Imagine a string pulling the crown of your head towards the sky
  - Walk with this elongated spine for 5 minutes
  - Pay attention to how this affects your mood and energy

Implement these posture adjustments throughout your day. Set reminders to check and correct your posture every hour.

By integrating these embodied practices into your daily life, you can actively engage your body in managing depression symptoms. Remember that consistency is key – start with small, manageable sessions and gradually increase duration and frequency. These somatic approaches complement traditional treatments for depression and can contribute significantly to overall well-being and mood regulation.

Chapter 9:

Mindfulness and Body-Centered Meditation

This chapter explores mindfulness practices that focus on bodily sensations to alleviate symptoms of anxiety and depression. These techniques enhance body awareness, promote relaxation, and cultivate a present-moment focus.

Body Scan Meditation

The body scan is a foundational practice in mindfulness that involves systematically focusing attention on different parts of the body. This technique helps increase body awareness, release tension, and promote relaxation.

Basic Body Scan Technique:
1. Lie down in a comfortable position, eyes closed.
2. Begin by focusing on your breath for a few moments.
3. Shift attention to your toes, noticing any sensations present.

4. Slowly move your focus up through your body, part by part:
     o Feet, ankles, calves, knees, thighs
     o Hips, lower back, abdomen, chest
     o Fingers, hands, arms, shoulders
     o Neck, face, scalp
5. For each body part, notice sensations without judgment.
6. If you encounter tension, breathe into that area, imagining the tension dissolving.
7. After reaching the top of your head, take a moment to feel your body as a whole.

Advanced Body Scan Practices:
1. Loving-Kindness Body Scan:
     o As you focus on each body part, silently offer it compassion and gratitude.
     o Use phrases like "May my feet be healthy and strong" or "I appreciate my hands for all they do."
2. Visualization-Enhanced Body Scan:
     o Imagine a warm, healing light moving through your body as you scan.
     o Visualize this light soothing and rejuvenating each body part.
3. Micro Body Scan:
     o Focus on smaller, often overlooked areas like individual fingers or facial muscles.
     o This heightened attention can reveal subtle tensions and promote deeper relaxation.

Aim to practice the body scan for 15-30 minutes daily. Consistency is key to experiencing the full benefits of this practice.

Mindful Walking

Mindful walking combines gentle physical activity with present-moment awareness. This practice can be particularly beneficial for those who find seated meditation challenging.

Basic Mindful Walking Technique:
1. Choose a safe path, indoors or outdoors.
2. Stand still, feeling your feet on the ground.
3. Begin walking at a slow, natural pace.
4. Focus on the sensations of walking:
   - The lifting of your foot
   - The movement through the air
   - The placing of your foot on the ground
5. When your mind wanders, gently bring attention back to the walking sensations.

Advanced Mindful Walking Practices:
1. Sensory Expansion:
   o Gradually expand your awareness to include other senses.
   o Notice sounds, smells, and visual input while maintaining focus on walking sensations.
2. Pace Variation:
   o Experiment with different walking speeds.

- o Notice how changes in pace affect your body and mind.
3. Terrain Awareness:
   - o Walk on various surfaces (grass, sand, pavement).
   - o Pay attention to how different terrains affect your balance and muscle engagement.
4. Emotional Check-In:
   - o As you walk, periodically scan your emotional state.
   - o Notice any connections between your emotions and physical sensations.

Practice mindful walking for 10-20 minutes daily, gradually increasing duration as you become more comfortable with the technique.

Somatic Mindfulness in Daily Life

Integrating body-centered mindfulness into everyday activities can significantly enhance overall well-being and stress management.

Practical Somatic Mindfulness Exercises:
1. Mindful Eating:
   - o Before eating, take three deep breaths.
   - o Notice the appearance, smell, and texture of your food.
   - o Chew slowly, savoring each bite.
   - o Pay attention to the sensations of swallowing and fullness.

2. Breath Awareness Breaks:
   o Set reminders throughout the day.
   o When prompted, take 3-5 mindful breaths.
   o Focus on the physical sensations of breathing in your body.
3. Posture Check-Ins:
   o Periodically scan your body posture throughout the day.
   o Notice any areas of tension or misalignment.
   o Make gentle adjustments to promote better alignment and ease.
4. Emotional Embodiment:
   o When you experience a strong emotion, pause.
   o Notice where you feel the emotion in your body.
   o Breathe into that area, allowing the sensation to be present without judgment.
5. Mindful Hand Washing:
   o Focus fully on the sensations of washing your hands.
   o Notice the temperature of the water, the texture of soap, and the movement of your hands.
6. Doorway Mindfulness:
   o Use doorways as mindfulness triggers.
   o Each time you pass through a door, take a conscious breath and notice your body.
7. Tech Use Body Awareness:
   o When using devices, periodically check your body posture.

- Notice any tension in your neck, shoulders, or hands.
- Take brief stretching breaks to release accumulated tension.

Implement these practices gradually, starting with one or two that resonate with you. Over time, expand your repertoire of somatic mindfulness techniques.

By consistently engaging in these body-centered mindfulness practices, you can develop a deeper connection with your physical self, reduce stress, and enhance overall well-being. Remember that mindfulness is a skill that improves with practice. Be patient and compassionate with yourself as you cultivate these new habits.

Chapter 10:

Emotional Regulation through the Body

This chapter explores somatic approaches to emotional regulation, focusing on techniques that use bodily awareness and physical interventions to manage and process emotions effectively.

Naming and Locating Emotions in the Body

Developing the ability to identify and locate emotions within the body is a crucial step in emotional regulation. This practice, often called "embodied emotional awareness," enhances emotional intelligence and provides a foundation for effective self-management.

Emotional Body Mapping Exercise:
1. Obtain a blank outline of a human body or draw one yourself.
2. Reflect on a recent emotional experience.
3. Ask yourself: "Where do I feel this emotion in my body?"

4. Use colors or shading to mark these areas on the body outline.
5. Note the quality of the sensation (e.g., tight, warm, heavy, tingling).
6. Repeat this process for different emotions over time.

Advanced Practices:

1. Emotion-Sensation Journaling:
   - Keep a daily log of emotions and their corresponding physical sensations.
   - Note patterns and changes over time.
2. Real-Time Body Scanning:
   - When you notice an emotion arising, pause.
   - Conduct a quick body scan to locate the physical manifestation of the emotion.
   - Describe the sensation to yourself in detail.
3. Emotional Vocabulary Expansion:
   - Learn new emotion words (e.g., melancholy, exuberant, wistful).
   - Practice identifying these nuanced emotions in your body.
4. Partner Sharing:
   - Describe your embodied emotional experiences to a trusted friend or therapist.
   - This verbalization enhances awareness and processing.

Consistent practice of these techniques increases your ability to recognize and understand emotions as they arise, providing a crucial first step in regulation.

Self-Soothing Techniques

Self-soothing techniques engage the body's natural calming mechanisms, helping to regulate intense emotions and reduce stress.

Key Self-Soothing Practices:
1. Deep Pressure Stimulation:
   - Use a weighted blanket or apply firm pressure to large muscle groups.
   - This activates the parasympathetic nervous system, promoting calm.
2. Temperature Regulation:
   - Hold an ice pack to the back of your neck or splash cold water on your face to reduce intense emotions.
   - Use warmth (e.g., a heating pad) for comfort and relaxation.
3. Rhythmic Movement:
   - Engage in repetitive, rhythmic movements like rocking or swaying.
   - This can help regulate the nervous system and soothe intense emotions.
4. Self-Massage:
   - Gently massage your hands, feet, or temples.
   - Focus on the physical sensations to ground yourself.
5. Bilateral Stimulation:
   - Alternately tap your right and left knees or shoulders.

- This rhythmic, side-to-side stimulation can help process and regulate emotions.

6. Sensory Grounding:
   - Engage your senses with calming stimuli (e.g., lavender scent, soft textures).
   - Create a "sensory kit" with items that engage each sense positively.

7. Vagus Nerve Stimulation:
   - Practice humming, singing, or gargling to stimulate the vagus nerve.
   - This activates the parasympathetic nervous system, promoting relaxation.

Experiment with these techniques to find which work best for you in different emotional states. Create a personalized "emotional first-aid kit" with your preferred tools.

Anger Release Methods

Anger, when not properly expressed, can lead to physical and emotional distress. These somatic methods provide healthy outlets for anger, promoting release and regulation.

Effective Anger Release Techniques:

1. Progressive Muscle Relaxation for Anger:
   - Tense each muscle group forcefully while thinking of your anger.

o Release suddenly, imagining the anger leaving your body.

o Progress through all major muscle groups.

2. Controlled Physical Release:

o Punch a pillow or punching bag.

o Tear paper or squeeze stress balls.

o Focus on the physical sensation of release.

3. Power Poses:

o Adopt expansive, powerful body postures.

o Hold for 2 minutes while breathing deeply.

o This can help transform angry energy into a sense of personal power.

4. Primal Sound Release:

o In a private space, vocalize your anger through shouts or growls.

o Focus on the physical sensation of making these sounds.

5. Anger Dance:

o Put on intense music and dance out your anger.

o Let your movements express the emotion fully.

6. Writing and Ripping:

o Write your angry thoughts on paper.

o Physically tear up the paper, symbolically releasing the anger.

7. Mindful Anger Observation:

o Sit quietly and observe anger sensations in your body.

o Breathe into these areas without trying to change the feeling.

o Notice how the sensations shift and change over time.

Safety Note: Ensure you're in a safe environment when practicing these techniques. If anger is a persistent issue, consider working with a therapist specializing in anger management.

Integrating Emotional Regulation Practices:
1. Create an Emotion Regulation Plan:
    o List your common emotional triggers.
    o Identify which techniques work best for each emotion.
    o Keep this plan easily accessible for quick reference.
2. Daily Body-Emotion Check-Ins:
    o Set regular times for brief body scans and emotional check-ins.
    o This builds the habit of embodied emotional awareness.
3. Preventative Practice:
    o Engage in calming somatic practices daily, not just during emotional intensity.
    o This builds resilience and makes regulation easier during challenging times.
4. Combine Techniques:
    o Experiment with combining different methods (e.g., temperature regulation with bilateral stimulation).
    o Find synergistic combinations that work best for you.

By consistently practicing these somatic emotional regulation techniques, you can develop greater emotional resilience and self-awareness. Remember that emotional regulation is a skill that improves with practice. Be patient and compassionate with yourself as you develop these abilities. Over time, you'll find that you have a robust toolkit for managing a wide range of emotional experiences through your body.

PART III:

SOMATIC THERAPY FOR STRESS AND BURNOUT

This section focuses on the application of somatic therapy to address the pervasive issues of chronic stress and burnout. In our fast-paced world, these conditions have become increasingly common, taking a toll on both physical and mental health.

We'll explore how stress and burnout manifest in the body, the impact on the nervous system, and somatic techniques for prevention and recovery. This part covers embodied stress management, somatic resourcing, and practices for restoring vitality. Through practical exercises and real-life examples, you'll learn how to use somatic awareness to recognize early signs of stress, build resilience, and cultivate a sustainable balance between activity and rest in your daily life.

Chapter 11:

Recognizing Stress and Burnout in the Body

This chapter focuses on identifying the physical manifestations of chronic stress and burnout. Understanding these bodily signals is crucial for early intervention and effective management of stress-related issues.

Physical Signs of Chronic Stress

Chronic stress can have profound effects on the body, often manifesting in various physical symptoms. Recognizing these signs is the first step in addressing stress-related issues:

1. Muscular Tension:
   - Persistent tightness in neck, shoulders, and jaw
   - Frequent headaches or migraines
   - Lower back pain
2. Digestive Disturbances:
   - Stomach ulcers or persistent indigestion
   - Irritable bowel syndrome (IBS)
   - Changes in appetite (increase or decrease)
3. Cardiovascular Changes:

- o Elevated blood pressure
- o Increased heart rate
- o Palpitations or chest pain
4. Sleep Disruptions:
   - o Difficulty falling asleep or staying asleep
   - o Waking up feeling unrefreshed
   - o Excessive daytime fatigue
5. Skin Issues:
   - o Acne breakouts
   - o Eczema flare-ups
   - o Excessive sweating
6. Immune System Suppression:
   - o Frequent colds or infections
   - o Slow wound healing
   - o Reactivation of dormant viruses (e.g., herpes)
7. Hormonal Imbalances:
   - o Irregular menstrual cycles
   - o Decreased libido
   - o Thyroid dysfunction
8. Neurological Symptoms:
   - o Difficulty concentrating or brain fog
   - o Memory problems
   - o Dizziness or vertigo

Stress Awareness Exercise:
- Conduct a daily body scan, noting areas of tension or discomfort
- Keep a log of physical symptoms and their intensity
- Look for patterns in symptom occurrence and potential stress triggers

Burnout Symptoms and Stages

Burnout is a state of physical, emotional, and mental exhaustion caused by prolonged exposure to high levels of stress. It develops gradually, often in stages:

Stage 1: Honeymoon Phase
- High job satisfaction and energy
- Commitment to work responsibilities
- Occasional stress symptoms begin to appear

Physical signs:
- Mild fatigue after work
- Occasional headaches
- Minor sleep disturbances

Stage 2: Onset of Stress
- Job satisfaction decreases
- Work efficiency declines
- Sleep disturbances increase

Physical signs:
- Frequent headaches
- Muscle tension
- Digestive issues

Stage 3: Chronic Stress
- Persistent tiredness
- Procrastination increases
- Physical symptoms intensify

Physical signs:
- Chronic fatigue
- Persistent muscle pain

- Changes in eating habits

Stage 4: Burnout
- Self-doubt and feeling of failure set in
- Desire to "escape" from responsibilities
- Physical symptoms become severe

Physical signs:
- Chronic headaches or migraines
- Gastrointestinal disorders
- Significant changes in sleep patterns

Stage 5: Habitual Burnout
- Burnout symptoms become embedded in daily life
- Significant physical and emotional problems may develop

Physical signs:
- Chronic mental and physical fatigue
- Potential development of stress-related illnesses (e.g., cardiovascular disease, depression)

Burnout Self-Assessment:
- Rate your energy levels daily (1-10 scale)
- Note changes in sleep patterns and quality
- Track frequency and intensity of physical symptoms
- Observe changes in work attitude and performance

The Allostatic Load Concept

Allostatic load refers to the cumulative wear and tear on the body's systems due to chronic stress. This concept helps explain how prolonged stress can lead to various health problems.

Key Components of Allostatic Load:
1. Primary Mediators:
   - Stress hormones (e.g., cortisol, adrenaline)
   - Pro-inflammatory cytokines
2. Secondary Outcomes:
   - Metabolic changes (e.g., elevated blood sugar, cholesterol)
   - Cardiovascular alterations (e.g., increased blood pressure)
3. Tertiary Outcomes:
   - Chronic diseases (e.g., diabetes, heart disease)
   - Cognitive decline
   - Accelerated aging

How Allostatic Load Accumulates:
1. Frequent Stress Activation:
   - Repeated activation of stress response systems
   - Inadequate recovery time between stressors
2. Failed Shutdown:
   - Difficulty "turning off" stress responses
   - Persistent elevated stress hormones
3. Inadequate Response:
   - Insufficient stress response to meet demands

o Can lead to compensatory hyperactivation of other systems
4. Lack of Adaptation:
   o Failure to habituate to repeated stressors
   o Results in prolonged stress responses

Measuring Allostatic Load:
- Biomarkers: Cortisol levels, blood pressure, waist-hip ratio
- Subjective measures: Stress perception scales, quality of life assessments

Allostatic Load Reduction Strategies:
1. Stress Management Techniques:
   o Regular meditation or mindfulness practice
   o Time management and prioritization skills
2. Lifestyle Modifications:
   o Consistent sleep schedule
   o Balanced nutrition
   o Regular physical exercise
3. Social Support:
   o Cultivating supportive relationships
   o Seeking professional help when needed
4. Recovery Practices:
   o Implementing daily relaxation techniques
   o Taking regular breaks during work
5. Environmental Adjustments:
   o Creating a stress-reduced living and working space
   o Setting boundaries to reduce exposure to stressors

Understanding Allostatic Load empowers individuals to take proactive steps in managing stress and preventing burnout. By recognizing the cumulative nature of stress on the body, one can implement targeted interventions to reduce this load and improve overall health and resilience.

By developing awareness of the physical signs of chronic stress, understanding the stages of burnout, and recognizing the concept of allostatic load, individuals can take informed action to manage stress effectively.

Chapter 12:

Resetting the Nervous System

This chapter focuses on practical approaches to regulating the nervous system, drawing on cutting-edge neuroscience and time-tested somatic practices to alleviate stress and promote resilience.

Polyvagal Theory in Practice

Polyvagal Theory, developed by Dr. Stephen Porges, provides a framework for understanding the autonomic nervous system's role in our emotional states and social behavior. This theory identifies three distinct branches of the autonomic nervous system:

1. Ventral Vagal Complex (VVC): The "safe and social" state
2. Sympathetic Nervous System (SNS): The "fight or flight" state
3. Dorsal Vagal Complex (DVC): The "freeze" state

Understanding these states allows for targeted interventions:

VVC Activation Techniques:
- Deep, slow breathing
- Singing or humming
- Engaging in positive social interactions

SNS Regulation Methods:
- Progressive muscle relaxation
- Vigorous exercise followed by cool-down
- Bilateral stimulation (e.g., alternating hand taps)

DVC Deactivation Strategies:
- Gentle movement or stretching
- Focusing on external sensory inputs
- Gradual exposure to safe social engagement

Practical Polyvagal Exercise: State Shifting
1. Identify your current autonomic state
2. Choose an appropriate technique based on your state
3. Practice the technique for 5-10 minutes
4. Reassess your state and adjust as needed

Nervous System Regulation Techniques

These techniques aim to balance the autonomic nervous system, promoting a state of calm alertness.
1. Diaphragmatic Breathing:

- Place one hand on chest, one on abdomen
- Inhale deeply through the nose, expanding the abdomen
- Exhale slowly through pursed lips
- Practice for 5-10 minutes daily

2. Heart Rate Variability (HRV) Breathing:
   - Inhale for 4 counts, exhale for 6 counts
   - Maintain this 10-second cycle for 5 minutes
   - Use an HRV biofeedback device for enhanced results

3. Cold Exposure:
   - End showers with 30 seconds of cold water
   - Focus on calm, controlled breathing during exposure
   - Gradually increase duration over time

4. Grounding Techniques:
   - Walk barefoot on natural surfaces
   - Hold and manipulate textured objects
   - Practice the 5-4-3-2-1 sensory awareness exercise

5. Rhythmic Movement:
   - Engage in repetitive, bilateral movements (e.g., walking, swimming)
   - Focus on the rhythm and physical sensations
   - Practice for 15-30 minutes daily

6. Tension and Release:
   - Systematically tense and relax muscle groups
   - Hold tension for 5 seconds, release for 10 seconds
   - Progress from feet to head

7. Vagus Nerve Stimulation:

- Gently massage the area behind the ears
- Practice gargling or loud humming
- Use a specialized vagus nerve stimulation device (under professional guidance)

Nervous System Check-In Practice:
- Set reminders throughout the day
- When prompted, assess your current state (VVC, SNS, or DVC)
- Apply an appropriate regulation technique
- Note the effects in a journal

Sleep Hygiene and Somatic Practices

Quality sleep is crucial for nervous system regulation. These somatic practices enhance sleep hygiene:

1. Body Temperature Regulation:
   - Take a warm bath 1-2 hours before bedtime
   - Keep bedroom cool (60-67°F or 15-19°C)
   - Wear breathable, comfortable sleepwear
2. Progressive Muscle Relaxation for Sleep:
   - Lie in bed and tense each muscle group for 5 seconds
   - Release tension suddenly, focusing on the sensation of relaxation
   - Progress from toes to head
3. Pre-Sleep Somatic Routine:
   - Gentle stretching or yoga for 10-15 minutes
   - Focus on slow, deep breathing
   - End with a brief body scan meditation

4. Sleep Position Awareness:
   o Experiment with different sleep positions
   o Use pillows to support neutral spine alignment
   o Notice how different positions affect your sleep quality
5. Rhythmic Sleep Induction:
   o In bed, practice rhythmic breathing (4-7-8 technique)
   o Synchronize breath with gentle rocking or swaying
   o Continue until drowsiness sets in
6. Sensory Sleep Environment:
   o Use blackout curtains or an eye mask for darkness
   o Employ white noise or nature sounds if helpful
   o Choose bedding textures that feel soothing
7. Daytime Practices for Better Sleep:
   o Expose yourself to natural light upon waking
   o Engage in moderate exercise during the day
   o Practice stress-reduction techniques throughout the day

Sleep Hygiene Assessment:
- Keep a sleep diary for two weeks
- Note bedtime, wake time, and sleep quality
- Record pre-sleep activities and environmental factors
- Identify patterns and areas for improvement

Implementing these nervous system regulation techniques and sleep hygiene practices can significantly reduce stress and improve overall well-being. Consistency is key – aim to incorporate these practices into your daily routine for optimal results. Remember that individual responses may vary, so it's important to experiment and find the combination of techniques that works best for you.

By resetting your nervous system through these methods, you can build resilience against stress, improve your sleep quality, and enhance your overall capacity to handle life's challenges. Regular practice of these techniques can lead to lasting improvements in both physical and mental health.

Chapter 13:

Energy Management and Boundaries

This chapter explores somatic approaches to managing energy and establishing healthy boundaries, essential skills for preventing burnout and maintaining overall well-being.

Body-Based Time Management

Traditional time management often neglects the body's natural rhythms. Body-based time management aligns tasks with your energy levels and physical needs.

1. Circadian Rhythm Mapping:
   - Track your energy levels hourly for a week
   - Note times of peak alertness and fatigue
   - Schedule demanding tasks during high-energy periods

2. Ultradian Rhythm Integration:
   - Work in 90-minute focused sessions
   - Take 20-30 minute breaks between sessions
   - Use breaks for physical movement or relaxation

3. Body Clock Task Alignment:
   - Schedule creative work when body temperature is rising (typically morning)
   - Plan physical tasks for late afternoon when muscle strength peaks
   - Reserve evenings for low-key, relaxing activities
4. Energy Type Identification:
   - Determine if you're a "lark" (morning person) or "owl" (night person)
   - Adjust your schedule to leverage your natural energy patterns
5. Physical Cues for Time Blocks:
   - Use postural changes to signal task transitions
   - Example: Sit for focused work, stand for brainstorming, walk for problem-solving
6. Somatic Productivity Techniques:
   - Implement the "Pomodoro Technique" with body awareness
   - During breaks, perform quick body scans or stretches
   - Use physical movement to reset between tasks
7. Energy Expense Budgeting:
   - Categorize tasks by energy expenditure (high, medium, low)
   - Balance your daily "energy budget" across these categories
   - Monitor physical signs of energy depletion and adjust accordingly

Body-Based Time Management Exercise:

- Create a weekly schedule based on your energy mapping
- Experiment with this schedule for two weeks
- Adjust based on your body's feedback and performance outcomes

Setting Energetic Boundaries

Energetic boundaries protect your physical and emotional well-being from external demands and influences.

1. Somatic Boundary Visualization:
   - Imagine a protective energy field surrounding your body
   - Visualize this field expanding or contracting based on your needs
   - Practice maintaining this field during interactions
2. Grounding for Boundary Setting:
   - Before entering challenging situations, practice a quick grounding exercise
   - Feel your feet firmly connected to the ground
   - Imagine roots growing from your feet, anchoring you
3. Body Language for Boundaries:
   - Practice assertive postures: stand tall, shoulders back, chin parallel to ground
   - Use hand gestures to physically indicate limits (e.g., palm out for "stop")

- Maintain appropriate personal space in interactions

4. Energetic Cleansing Rituals:
   - Develop a post-interaction ritual to "clear" absorbed energy
   - Examples: Brushing off your body, visualizing a cleansing shower of light
   - Perform deep exhales to release tension and others' energy

5. Sensory Overwhelm Prevention:
   - Identify your sensory thresholds (noise, light, touch, etc.)
   - Create a "sensory haven" for overstimulation recovery
   - Use noise-cancelling headphones or sunglasses when needed

6. Emotional Contagion Awareness:
   - Notice when you're absorbing others' emotions
   - Practice "emotional differentiation" – distinguish your feelings from others'
   - Use physical cues (e.g., hand on heart) to center in your own experience

7. Digital Boundary Setting:
   - Create physical spaces free from digital devices
   - Set specific body-based cues for technology use (e.g., only check email while standing)
   - Practice regular "digital detox" periods, focusing on physical sensations

Energetic Boundary Exercise:
- In various interactions, notice your energy levels before and after
- Identify energy-draining vs. energy-enhancing encounters
- Implement appropriate boundary techniques in challenging situations

Saying "No" with Your Whole Self

Effective boundary-setting involves aligning your verbal and non-verbal communication.

1. Embodied "No" Practice:
   - Stand with feet hip-width apart, feel your connection to the ground
   - Take a deep breath, expanding your chest
   - Say "No" while extending one hand, palm out
   - Notice the sensations in your body as you do this
2. Congruence Check:
   - Before responding to requests, pause and check in with your body
   - Notice any tension, contraction, or expansion
   - Ensure your verbal response matches your physical sensations
3. Boundary Assertion Roleplay:
   - Practice saying "No" to common requests with a partner
   - Focus on maintaining aligned posture and clear tone

o Debrief on the physical sensations experienced

4. Delayed Response Technique:
   o When faced with a request, state that you'll "check your schedule"
   o Use this time to consult your body's wisdom
   o Respond later with a grounded "Yes" or "No"
5. Physical Cues for Overcommitment:
   o Identify your body's signals of overextension (e.g., shoulder tension, shallow breathing)
   o Use these as cues to reassess commitments and say "No" when necessary
6. Compassionate Refusal Practice:
   o Develop a script for kind but firm refusals
   o Practice delivering these while maintaining an open, relaxed posture
   o Focus on expressing empathy while holding your ground
7. Post-Refusal Self-Care:
   o After saying "No," especially if it's challenging, engage in a nurturing physical activity
   o This reinforces that boundary-setting is self-care, not selfishness

Whole-Self "No" Exercise:
- Identify a situation where you need to say "No"
- Practice your response using the embodied techniques
- Deliver your "No" and immediately afterward, note your physical sensations

- Reflect on the experience and adjust your approach as needed

By integrating these body-based approaches to time management, energetic boundaries, and assertive communication, you can significantly enhance your ability to manage stress and prevent burnout. Remember, these skills develop with practice. Be patient with yourself and celebrate small improvements as you cultivate a more balanced, boundary-aware lifestyle.

Chapter 14:

Somatic Self-Care Rituals

Somatic self-care rituals are essential practices that help integrate body awareness and healing into our daily lives. These rituals serve as anchors, allowing us to consistently reconnect with our bodies and maintain the benefits of somatic therapy. This chapter explores various somatic self-care rituals, including morning and evening routines, micro-breaks throughout the day, and weekend reset practices.

Morning and Evening Routines

Morning Routine:

A somatic morning routine sets a positive tone for the day, helping to awaken the body and cultivate mindfulness from the start.

1. Body Scan Upon Waking: Begin your day with a gentle body scan while still in bed. Move your attention slowly from your toes to the crown of your head, noticing any sensations without judgment. This practice helps transition from sleep to wakefulness while promoting body awareness.

2. Mindful Stretching: Engage in 5-10 minutes of gentle stretching, focusing on areas that feel tense

or contracted. Pay close attention to the sensations of muscles lengthening and joints moving. This not only improves physical flexibility but also enhances your mind-body connection.

3. Grounding Exercise: Stand barefoot on the floor or, if possible, on grass outside. Feel the connection between your feet and the ground. Imagine roots growing from your feet into the earth, anchoring you. This practice promotes a sense of stability and connection to your environment.

4. Mindful Hygiene Practices: Transform your morning hygiene routine into a somatic experience. While brushing your teeth, focus on the sensations in your mouth. During your shower, pay attention to the feeling of water on your skin and the scents of your toiletries.

Evening Routine:

An evening somatic routine helps transition from the activities of the day to a state of relaxation, promoting better sleep and overall well-being.

1. Progressive Muscle Relaxation: Lie down comfortably and systematically tense and relax each muscle group in your body, starting from your toes and moving upward. This practice releases accumulated physical tension and prepares the body for rest.

2. Breath-Focused Meditation: Spend 5-10 minutes focusing on your breath. Notice the sensation of air moving in and out of your nostrils or the rise

and fall of your chest or abdomen. This calms the nervous system and promotes mental clarity.

3. Gentle Yoga or Stretching: Engage in gentle yoga poses or stretches that focus on releasing tension in areas that tend to hold stress, such as the neck, shoulders, and lower back. Move slowly and mindfully, synchronizing movement with breath.

4. Body Gratitude Practice: Before sleep, mentally scan your body and express gratitude for different parts and their functions. This fosters a positive relationship with your body and can improve body image and self-esteem.

Micro-breaks Throughout the Day

Incorporating brief somatic practices throughout your day helps maintain body awareness and manage stress. These micro-breaks can be as short as 1-2 minutes and can be easily integrated into a busy schedule.

1. Posture Check-ins: Set reminders to check your posture every hour. Notice any areas of tension or misalignment and make gentle adjustments. This prevents the accumulation of physical stress and promotes better body awareness.

2. Mindful Walking: When moving between tasks or locations, practice mindful walking. Feel the sensation of your feet touching the ground, the movement of your legs, and the swing of your

arms. This grounds you in the present moment and provides a brief respite from mental activity.

3. Three-Breath Reset: Take three conscious, deep breaths whenever you feel stressed or overwhelmed. Focus on the sensation of the breath moving in and out of your body. This simple practice activates the parasympathetic nervous system, promoting calm and focus.

4. Desk Stretches: If you work at a desk, incorporate brief stretching sequences. Focus on areas prone to tension like the neck, shoulders, and wrists. These stretches not only relieve physical discomfort but also serve as moments of somatic awareness.

5. Emotional Check-ins: Pause briefly to notice your emotional state and where you feel it in your body. This practice enhances emotional awareness and can prevent the buildup of unexpressed feelings.

Weekend Reset Practices

Weekends offer an opportunity for more extended somatic self-care practices that reset and rejuvenate your mind-body system.

1. Nature Immersion: Spend time in nature, engaging all your senses. Feel the texture of tree bark, listen to bird songs, smell the scents of plants. This practice, known as "forest bathing" in Japan, has been shown to reduce stress and improve overall well-being.

2. Extended Body Scan Meditation: Dedicate 20-30 minutes to a comprehensive body scan meditation. This deeper practice allows for more nuanced awareness of bodily sensations and can reveal areas of chronic tension or holding patterns.

3. Expressive Movement: Engage in free-form movement or dance without judgment. Allow your body to move intuitively, expressing emotions and releasing tension. This practice fosters creativity and emotional release through physical expression.

4. Somatic Journaling: Spend time writing about your physical sensations, emotions, and any insights gained from your somatic practices throughout the week. This reflection deepens your understanding of your mind-body patterns and tracks your progress over time.

5. Sensory Exploration: Dedicate time to fully exploring one of your senses. For example, mindfully prepare and eat a meal, focusing on tastes and textures. Or listen to music with your full attention, noticing how different sounds affect your body. This heightens sensory awareness and deepens your connection to the present moment.

6. Restorative Yoga or Self-Massage: Practice restorative yoga poses using props to fully support your body, allowing for deep relaxation. Alternatively, engage in self-massage, using techniques like foam rolling or gentle self-touch to release tension and promote body awareness.

Implementing these somatic self-care rituals consistently can significantly enhance your overall well-being, deepen your mind-body connection, and provide practical tools for managing stress and emotions. Remember to approach these practices with curiosity and compassion, allowing your experience to unfold naturally without judgment or expectation.

Chapter 15:

Reconnecting with Joy and Purpose

In this chapter, we explore how somatic practices can help us rediscover joy and purpose in our lives. We'll examine the role of pleasure in combating burnout, learn techniques for embodied goal-setting, and discover how somatic awareness can align our actions with our core values.

Pleasure as an Antidote to Burnout

Burnout, characterized by emotional exhaustion, detachment, and reduced efficacy, often disconnects us from our bodies and the simple pleasures of life. Reintroducing pleasure through somatic practices can be a powerful tool for recovery and prevention.
Understanding Pleasure from a Somatic Perspective:
In somatic therapy, pleasure isn't just about fleeting enjoyment. It's a deep, embodied experience that activates the parasympathetic nervous system, promoting relaxation, healing, and overall well-being.

Techniques for Cultivating Pleasure:

1. Sensory Engagement: Dedicate time each day to fully engage with pleasurable sensory experiences. This might involve:
   - Savoring a favorite food, focusing on its taste, texture, and aroma
   - Listening to music that moves you, noticing how it affects your body
   - Touching different textures and observing the sensations they produce

2. Movement for Joy: Engage in movement solely for the pleasure it brings, without focus on fitness goals. This could include:
   - Dancing freely to music you love
   - Stretching in ways that feel good to your body
   - Exploring gentle, flowing movements like Tai Chi or Qigong

3. Mindful Rest: Practice restorative poses or activities that allow deep relaxation. For example:
   - Lie in a comfortable position and scan your body for areas of tension, consciously releasing them
   - Practice progressive muscle relaxation, tensing and then releasing each muscle group
   - Use weighted blankets or soft textures to stimulate the body's relaxation response

4. Nature Connection: Spend time in nature, using all your senses to absorb its rejuvenating effects:

- Walk barefoot on grass or sand, feeling the texture beneath your feet
- Sit quietly in a natural setting, listening to the sounds around you
- Observe the intricate details of plants or clouds, appreciating their beauty

Implementing Pleasure Practices:
Start by scheduling short "pleasure breaks" throughout your day. Even five minutes of focused, pleasurable activity can shift your nervous system state and combat burnout symptoms.

Embodied Goal-Setting

Traditional goal-setting often neglects the body's wisdom. Embodied goal-setting integrates somatic awareness into the process, leading to more authentic and sustainable objectives.

Steps for Embodied Goal-Setting:
1. Somatic Check-In: Before setting goals, conduct a body scan to assess your current state. Notice areas of tension, energy, or emptiness. This awareness can provide valuable information about your true needs and desires.
2. Visualize and Feel: As you consider potential goals, visualize achieving them. Pay close attention to how your body responds. Does it feel expansive and energized, or contracted and tense?

Your body's reaction can indicate whether a goal truly aligns with your deeper self.

3. Embody Your Future Self: Imagine yourself having achieved your goal. How does this future self move, stand, and breathe? Practice embodying these qualities in the present moment. This can build confidence and provide a somatic blueprint for progress.

4. Set Somatic Milestones: Alongside traditional milestones, establish somatic markers of progress. For example, if your goal is to reduce stress, a somatic milestone might be noticing your shoulders relaxing more easily or your breath becoming deeper.

5. Regular Body Check-Ins: As you work towards your goals, regularly check in with your body. Are you holding tension? Does pursuing the goal deplete or energize you? Use this information to adjust your approach or even reevaluate the goal itself.

Aligning Actions with Values through Somatic Awareness

Our bodies often signal when our actions are out of alignment with our core values. Developing somatic awareness can help us recognize and correct this misalignment.

Techniques for Somatic Value Alignment:

1. Identify Somatic Value Signatures: Reflect on your core values (e.g., honesty, compassion, creativity). For each value, recall times when you fully embodied it. Notice how your body felt in those moments. These somatic signatures can serve as guides for future decisions.

2. Decision-Making Body Scan: When faced with a decision, take a moment to check in with your body:
   - Take a few deep breaths to center yourself
   - Imagine choosing each option and notice your body's response
   - Pay attention to sensations like expansion, contraction, warmth, or tension
   - Use these bodily cues to inform your decision

3. Somatic Integrity Practices: Develop daily practices to strengthen your connection to your values:
   - Start your day by embodying a core value. If 'courage' is important to you, adopt a strong, open posture and feel the sensation of bravery in your body
   - Throughout the day, pause to ask, "How aligned do I feel right now?" Notice where and how you feel this in your body
   - When you notice misalignment, take a moment to adjust your posture, breath, or actions to realign with your values

4. Values-Based Movement: Create a movement sequence that represents your core values. This could be a series of gestures or a short dance. Practice this sequence regularly as a physical reminder of your values and to reinforce their embodiment.

5. Somatic Journaling: At the end of each day, reflect on moments when you felt most aligned with your values. Describe not just the situations, but also the bodily sensations associated with them. Over time, this practice will deepen your awareness of how value alignment feels in your body.

Implementing these somatic practices for reconnecting with joy and purpose can lead to a more authentic, fulfilling life. By tuning into your body's wisdom, you can set meaningful goals, make aligned decisions, and cultivate a deeper sense of pleasure and purpose in your daily experiences. Remember, this is a process of exploration and discovery. Be patient with yourself and approach these practices with curiosity and compassion.

Conclusion

Integrating Somatic Practices into Daily Life

As we conclude this exploration of somatic therapy, it's crucial to recognize that true transformation occurs through consistent, mindful integration of these practices into our daily lives. The journey of embodied healing is not a destination but a continuous process of self-discovery and growth.

Begin by incorporating small somatic moments throughout your day. This might involve brief body scans during work breaks, mindful breathing while commuting, or conscious movement as you transition between tasks. Over time, these micro-practices will cultivate a deeper awareness of your body's signals and needs.

Gradually expand your somatic repertoire, experimenting with different techniques to find what resonates most with you. Remember that what works best may change over time, so remain open and adaptable in your practice.

Create a supportive environment for your somatic journey. This might involve designating a quiet space for practice, setting reminders to check in with your body, or enlisting the support of friends or family members who understand the importance of your somatic work.

When to Seek Professional Help

While this book provides a comprehensive introduction to somatic therapy and offers numerous self-help techniques, it's important to recognize when professional guidance is necessary.

Consider seeking help from a qualified somatic therapist if:

1. You're dealing with severe trauma or deep-seated emotional issues that feel overwhelming to address on your own.
2. You experience persistent physical symptoms that don't resolve with self-practice.
3. You find yourself stuck in patterns of behavior or emotion that you can't seem to shift despite consistent effort.
4. You're facing a major life transition or crisis and feel you need additional support.
5. You're interested in diving deeper into somatic work and want personalized guidance to enhance your practice.

A professional can provide tailored strategies, offer a safe space for processing difficult emotions, and help you navigate challenges that arise during your somatic journey.

Embarking on the path of somatic therapy is a profound commitment to self-discovery and healing. It's a journey that invites you to listen deeply to your body's wisdom, to honor its messages, and to cultivate a more integrated sense of self.

As you continue on this path, remember that healing is not linear. There will be moments of breakthrough and clarity, as well as times of challenge and uncertainty. Approach each experience with curiosity and compassion, recognizing that every sensation, emotion, and insight is a valuable part of your journey.

Embodied healing extends far beyond individual well-being. As you become more attuned to your own body and emotions, you'll likely find that your relationships with others and with the world around you begin to shift. You may experience greater empathy, improved communication, and a deeper sense of connection to your environment.

Moreover, the skills you develop through somatic practice—such as self-regulation, mindful awareness, and embodied presence—can enhance every aspect of your life. From improving your performance at work to enriching your personal relationships, the benefits of somatic awareness ripple outward in countless ways.

As you close this book, remember that you've only just begun to tap into the vast potential of somatic healing. Continue to explore, to practice, and to grow. Trust in your body's innate wisdom and its capacity for healing. And above all, approach this journey with patience, curiosity, and an open heart.

Your body holds the key to profound healing and transformation. By committing to this path of embodied awareness, you're not just changing your own life—you're contributing to a larger shift towards a more embodied, empathetic, and connected world.

May your somatic journey be one of deep healing, joyful discovery, and transformative growth.

Glossary of Terms

1. **Autonomic Nervous System (ANS):** The part of the nervous system responsible for controlling involuntary bodily functions, including heart rate, digestion, respiratory rate, and arousal.
2. **Body Scan:** A mindfulness technique involving systematically focusing attention on different parts of the body, often used to increase body awareness and reduce tension.
3. **Embodiment:** The practice of fully inhabiting one's body and being aware of bodily sensations, emotions, and experiences in the present moment.
4. **Felt Sense:** A bodily sensation that has meaning; an internal bodily awareness that holds information about a situation, person, or event.
5. **Grounding:** Techniques used to bring one's attention to the present moment and to the body's connection with its environment, often used to reduce anxiety or overwhelm.
6. **Interoception:** The sense of the internal state of the body; the ability to perceive bodily sensations.
7. **Neuroception:** The subconscious system for detecting threats and safety, introduced by Stephen Porges as part of the Polyvagal Theory.
8. **Parasympathetic Nervous System:** The branch of the autonomic nervous system responsible for "rest and digest" functions, promoting calm and relaxation.

9. **Polyvagal Theory:** Developed by Stephen Porges, this theory describes the evolution and function of the autonomic nervous system and its role in social engagement, fight-or-flight, and freeze responses.
10. **Proprioception:** The senses of the relative position of one's own body parts and the strength of effort being employed in movement.
11. **Regulation:** The ability to manage and modify one's emotional and physiological states.
12. **Resourcing:** The practice of connecting with internal or external sources of support and strength to increase resilience and coping capacity.
13. **Somatic Experiencing:** A body-oriented approach to healing trauma and other stress disorders, developed by Peter Levine.
14. **Somatic Marker:** A physiological sensation associated with an emotion, used by the body and brain to guide decision-making.
15. **Sympathetic Nervous System:** The branch of the autonomic nervous system responsible for the "fight or flight" response, activating the body's stress response.
16. **Titration:** The processes of approaching difficult material or sensations in small, manageable amounts to avoid overwhelm.
17. **Tracking:** The practice of observing and following internal sensations, emotions, and thoughts as they change over time.

18. **Trauma Release Exercises (TRE):** A series of exercises that assist the body in releasing deep muscular patterns of stress, tension, and trauma.

19. **Vagus Nerve:** The main nerve of the parasympathetic nervous system, playing a crucial role in regulating various bodily functions and the stress response.

20. **Window of Tolerance:** The optimal zone of arousal in which a person is able to function most effectively. When we are within our window of tolerance, we can respond to life's stresses without becoming overwhelmed.